Causes of Cardiac Arrest

&

Treatment

of

Heart Diseases

By

Samson Richard

TABLE OF CONTENTS

Introduction

Chapter 1

Heart Disease

*Heart disease types

*Causes of Heart Disease

*Risks for developing heart disease

*Heart disease signs and symptoms

Chapter 2

Changes in Lifestyle

*The Impact of Exercise and Diet on Heart Disease

*Handling heart disease-related stress and anxiety

*Heart disease, alcohol use, and smoking

Chapter 3

Medicines for Heart Health

*How drugs for treating the heart work

*medication side effects and hazards

Introduction

Myocardial infarction (MI), another name for a heart attack, is when blood flow to a portion of the heart is cut off, harming or killing the heart muscle. The accumulation of plaque in the coronary arteries, which deliver oxygen-rich blood to the heart, is the most frequent reason for a heart attack. A blood clot that forms when plaque in the arteries bursts can either fully or partially block blood flow to the heart.

Chest pain, shortness of breath, sweating, nausea, and other symptoms may result from this. *Untreated heart attacks can permanently damage the heart muscle, resulting in consequences like heart failure, irregular heartbeats, and even death.* Consequently, it's crucial to get medical help right away if you think you're experiencing a heart attack. The most exciting finding, however, is that heart tissue can be strengthened to be more resilient and better equipped to recover from a heart attack. The tissue of the heart might suffer long-term damage from heart attacks. This is critical because, following a heart attack, clogged coronary arteries trigger death in some heart muscle cells and prevent the damaged tissue from healing. The cardioprotective effect, which we weren't expecting to detect or even notice, is maybe the most interesting because it has the most potential to influence the future. This makes it harder to repair heart damage in adult humans.

Chapter 1

Heart Disease

**Heart disease types*

Heart disease comes in a variety of forms.

The most prevalent kind of heart illness is **(coronary artery disease (CAD)**, which happens when the arteries supplying blood to the heart narrow or are clogged.

When the heart beats too quickly, too slowly, or irregularly, it is said to have an *(arrhythmia).*

When the heart cannot pump enough blood to satisfy the body's demands, *(heart failure)* develops.

*(Heart valve disease)*This condition occurs when one or more of the heart's valves malfunction, restricting blood flow.

Birth defects in the heart are referred to as *(congenital heart Disease)*

(Cardiomyopathy) Heart muscle conditions that might make it more difficult for the heart to pump blood are referred to by this term.

*(Pericardial disease)*This condition develops when the pericardium, the sac that surrounds the heart, becomes inflamed or infected.

(**Aortic aneurysm**) The major artery in the body's largest bulges or weakens, posing a risk of rupture and life-threatening hemorrhage.

(**Myocarditis**) is an illness brought on by a virus or bacterium that causes the heart muscle to inflame?

It's crucial to remember that several of these ailments can coexist or have connections to one another. If you believe you or a loved one may be experiencing any heart disease symptoms, it is essential to get medical advice.

*Causes of Heart Disease

Cardiovascular illness, sometimes referred to as **heart disease**, can have several causes. Bad lifestyle decisions can result in high blood pressure, obesity, and high cholesterol levels, which raise the risk of heart disease. **Sedentary behavior, poor eating habits, smoking, and excessive alcohol** use are further examples.

(Family history) Your risk of developing heart disease is higher if someone in your family has the condition.

(Age and gender) Men are more likely than women to acquire heart disease, and the risk of heart disease rises with age.

(Medical problems) Heart disease is more likely to occur in people who have certain medical disorders, such as diabetes, high blood pressure, high cholesterol, and obesity.

(*Chronic stress*) By boosting blood pressure and cholesterol levels, chronic stress can raise the risk of heart disease.

(*Sleep apnea*) A problem in which breathing repeatedly stops and begins while a person is asleep might cause an irregular heartbeat and raise their risk of developing heart disease. *Certain treatments,* including chemotherapy agents and several hormonal birth control methods, can raise the risk of heart disease.

(Genetics) Heart disease risk can be raised by some hereditary disorders, such as familial hypercholesterolemia.

It's significant to note that many of these risk factors are interconnected, and treating one risk factor can assist in lowering the likelihood of developing all of the other risk factors.

Risks for developing heart disease

A range of diseases that affect the heart and blood arteries collectively are referred to as heart disease or cardiovascular illness. The probability of having heart disease can be increased by several risk factors.

One of the main risk factors for heart disease is *(high blood pressure)* Too much blood pressure can damage the arteries and put additional strain on the heart.

High LDL ("bad") cholesterol levels can cause arteries to constrict and reduce blood flow to the heart by causing plaque to accumulate in the arteries.

(Smoking) Chemicals in tobacco smoke can damage blood vessels and raise the risk of heart disease.

(Diabetes) Due to the long-term harm that high blood sugar levels can bring to blood vessels, people with diabetes are more likely to develop heart disease.

*(**Obesity**)* Being obese or overweight can raise your chance of developing heart disease by placing more strain on your heart and raising your risk of developing other risk factors like high blood pressure and diabetes.

*(**Physical inactivity**)* Heart disease can occur as a result of infrequent exercise.

*(**Unhealthy diet**)* The risk of heart disease can be raised by consuming a diet that is heavy in salt, sugar, and saturated and

trans fats. To lower the chance of developing heart disease, it is crucial to control these risk factors through lifestyle adjustments and, in some circumstances, medicines.

Heart disease signs and symptoms

The specific type of heart disease a person has, as well as how severe the condition is, can affect the symptoms of the disease. Yet, the following are a few typical signs of cardiac disease:

One of the most typical signs of heart disease is *(**discomfort or pain in the chest**). An uncomfortable tightness, pressure,* squeezing, or burning sensation in the chest may be experienced. It can also be felt in the shoulders, back, neck, jaw, and arms.

(Breathlessness) This symptom might happen when moving around or even while you're just sitting still. Wheezing or tightness in the chest may be present as well.

(Fatigue) Even with very light exercise, people with heart disease may feel weak or weary.

Suddenly rising up or while engaging in physical exercise might cause *(dizziness or lightheadedness)*

(Leg, ankle, or foot swelling) may be a symptom of fluid retention brought on by heart failure.

(Unusual heartbeat) Heart illness may cause the heart to beat excessively quickly, too slowly, or unpredictably. It is significant to highlight that, particularly in the early stages of the ailment, some persons with heart disease may not exhibit any symptoms. As a result, it's crucial to visit a doctor often for checkups or lookout for any heart disease symptoms.

Chapter 2

Changes in Lifestyle

The Impact of Exercise and Diet on Heart Disease

Exercise and diet are two essential aspects that significantly affect heart disease. The leading cause of mortality in the world is heart disease, sometimes referred to as *cardiovascular diseases* Atherosclerosis happens when a buildup of plaque in the artery walls causes blood flow to the heart and other regions of the body to become restricted. (*Here are some of the key factors that make food and exercise so crucial for avoiding heart disease*) Your heart health may be directly impacted by the food you eat. Your chance of getting heart disease can be raised by consuming a diet that is heavy in salt, added sweets, and saturated and trans fats. The risk of heart disease can be reduced, however, by eating a diet high in fruits, vegetables, whole grains, lean meats, and healthy fats. Frequent exercise helps strengthen your heart and increase blood flow, both of which are ways to promote heart health. In addition to lowering cholesterol and blood sugar, exercise also lowers blood pressure, which can all be risk factors for heart disease. To prevent heart disease, it's crucial to maintain a healthy weight. You may acquire and keep a healthy weight with the aid of both nutrition and exercise.

Exercise can also aid in lowering stress levels, which can increase the risk of heart disease. Also, by giving your body the resources it needs to function correctly, eating a nutritious diet might help lower stress levels. Diet and exercise are essential for avoiding heart disease, to sum up. A nutritious diet and consistent exercise can help you maintain good heart health and lower your risk of heart disease.

***Handling heart disease-related stress and anxiety**

People with heart disease must learn to manage their stress and anxiety since these factors can aggravate pre-existing cardiac disorders and raise the chance of developing new ones. Stress and anxiety can be lessened by *using relaxation techniques including deep breathing, meditation, and yoga.* Stress and anxiety can be effectively reduced by exercise. Moreover, it may enhance cardiovascular health. It's crucial to get adequate sleep for general health, including heart health. Strive for **7-8 hours** of sleep every night, **minimum.** Consuming a **nutritious diet** reduced in **cholesterol, salt**, and **saturated** and **trans fats** can help reduce the risk of heart disease and enhance general health. **Stress and anxiety** can be lessened with the social *support of friends and family.* Think about getting **professional assistance** from a *mental health* expert if stress and worry are interfering with your everyday life. When recommended, take the prescribed medicine. Make sure to follow your doctor's instructions when taking any heart disease drugs that have been recommended to you. *In general, controlling stress and anxiety* is crucial to controlling cardiac disease. You may contribute to the improvement of your heart health and general well-being by implementing these techniques into your everyday practice.

*Heart disease, alcohol use, and smoking

Heart disease risk can be significantly decreased by giving up smoking and drinking less alcohol. Smoking destroys the blood vessel lining, raises blood pressure, and encourages plaque accumulation in the arteries, making it a major contributor to heart disease. People can lower their risk of heart disease and other illnesses including lung cancer, stroke, and chronic obstructive pulmonary disease by giving up *smoking (**COPD**)*. Alcohol intake can be decreased while still benefiting heart health. While moderate alcohol use (up to one drink per day for women and up to two drinks per day for men) may have some positive health effects, excessive alcohol use can raise your risk of high blood pressure, heart failure, and stroke. People can minimize their chance of developing these illnesses and enhance their general heart health by cutting back on or quitting drinking. Other lifestyle modifications that can improve heart health in addition to giving up smoking and consuming less alcohol include eating a balanced diet, maintaining a healthy weight, engaging in regular exercise, controlling stress, and getting adequate sleep. It's crucial to address these changes with a healthcare provider as well as any worries or inquiries you may have regarding your heart health.

Chapter 3

Medicines for Heart Health

*How drugs for treating the heart work

To treat cardiac disorders, a variety of treatments are available. The precise drug administered will depend on the ailment being treated as well as personal patient variables. These are some typical ways that medicines treat the heart,

Anticoagulants, commonly referred to as (**blood thinners**), prevent blood clots from developing in the heart's blood arteries. They lessen the possibility of heart attack, stroke, and other issues brought on by blood clots.

(Beta-blockers) Beta-blockers function by preventing the hormone adrenaline's effects, which can raise blood pressure and heart rate. Beta-blockers can

lower blood pressure, lessen the strain on the heart, and minimize the risk of heart attack by lowering these side effects.

(*ACE inhibitors*) ACE inhibitors function by preventing the hormone angiotensin II from constricting blood vessels and raising blood pressure. ACE inhibitors can decrease blood pressure and lessen the strain on the heart by inhibiting this hormone.

(Calcium channel blockers) Calcium channel blockers function by preventing the entry of calcium into the heart and blood vessel muscle cells. This aids in blood vessel relaxation, blood pressure reduction, and improved cardiac blood flow.

(Diuretics) Diuretics, sometimes referred to as water pills, increase the body's excretion of salt and water. This may assist in lowering blood pressure and lessening the

strain on the heart by reducing the amount of blood in the body.

(**Statins**) Statins function by inhibiting a liver enzyme involved in the production of cholesterol. Statins lower blood cholesterol levels, which lowers the risk of heart attack and stroke.

Overall, drugs may improve blood flow, lower blood pressure, lessen the burden on the heart, and prevent blood clots to treat cardiac diseases.

It's crucial to understand that the precise prescriptions provided will depend on the patient's individual medical history and condition, and should be reviewed with a healthcare expert.

medication side effects and hazards

Every drug has the possibility of adverse effects. *Headaches, tiredness, nausea, and dizziness* are a few typical adverse effects. Nevertheless, more severe side effects like allergic responses, respiratory problems, and variations in heart rate or blood pressure can also happen.

The following are possible additional dangers of pharmaceutical use

(**Drug interactions**) Certain medicines may have undesirable effects or lessen the efficiency of one or both medicines when used with other medicines, vitamins, or dietary supplements.

An (overdose) can result in major health issues or even death if a medicine is taken in excess.

(Addiction or dependency) If used often or in large doses, some drugs can become addictive or cause dependence.

(Birth problems) Taking some drugs while pregnant might result in birth defects.

(Damage to the liver or kidneys) Certain drugs have the potential to harm your liver or kidneys,

particularly if you take them often or in excessive amounts.

(Blood disorders) Some drugs may have an impact on the synthesis of blood cells, which may result in anemia, bleeding issues, or a higher risk of infection.

Always read the drug label and pay close attention to the directions. See your healthcare practitioner if you notice any adverse effects or have questions regarding your medicine.

Chapter 4

Medical Methods for Heart Wellness

**Angioplasty and stenting for the heart*

Medical techniques such as **coronary angioplasty and stenting** are used to treat **coronary artery disease** (**CAD**), a condition in which the arteries that supply blood to the heart narrow or become clogged as a result of plaque accumulation.

Chest discomfort (angina), breathlessness, heart attacks, and other consequences might result from this. A short, flexible tube known as ***a catheter*** is introduced into an ***artery*** in the ***groin or arm*** and directed to the ***heart's blocked*** or ***constricting artery*** during ***coronary angioplasty***. To open up the artery and increase blood flow to the heart, a little balloon at the end of the catheter is inflated. To assist keep the artery open, a stent *(a tiny mesh tube)* may occasionally be placed within it. Blood can flow more freely to the heart since the stent is permanently inserted into the artery. A *tiny incision* and a speedy recovery are the hallmarks of minimally invasive procedures like coronary angioplasty and stenting, which are frequently carried out under local anesthetic. *They are frequently used as a post-operative procedure or to address artery blockages that are not severe enough to necessitate bypass surgery.* Although angioplasty and stenting are often regarded as safe and successful procedures, there are potential dangers and side *effects, including bleeding, infection, blood clots, and arterial* or *surrounding tissue damage.* Your doctor will assess your unique situation and advise on the best course of action for you.

Cardiovascular artery bypass grafting

One type of surgical technique used to treat coronary artery disease is **coronary artery bypass grafting (CABG) (CAD)**. By grafting a healthy blood vessel from another region of the body onto the restricted or obstructed coronary artery, a surgeon can establish a new conduit for blood to flow to the heart. To reach the heart during **CABG**, the patient is given general anesthesia, and the surgeon creates a chest incision. Afterward, the surgeon makes a new route for blood to flow to the heart by grafting a healthy blood vessel onto the blocked or restricted coronary artery, such as the internal mammary artery or a vein from the leg. Patients with severe CAD who have not responded to other therapies, such as drugs or lifestyle modifications, often undergo CABG. Moreover, it might be used as a last resort for unstable angina or cardiac attacks.

The patient will need to relax and refrain from the heavy activity for several weeks after the surgery, during which time they will typically be monitored in the hospital for several days. Most patients who receive CABG may anticipate seeing a considerable improvement in their symptoms and quality of life with the right treatment and supervision.

Heart valve replacement

One or more of the heart valves can be repaired or replaced by a surgical procedure called heart valve surgery. Four valves of the heart assist in controlling blood flow throughout the body. These valves include the aortic, mitral, tricuspid, and pulmonary valves. When one or more of these valves develop damage or illness and can no longer function effectively, heart valve surgery is typically advised. **Valve stenosis (narrowing** *of the valve)*, *valve regurgitation (blood flowing through the valve)*, and *valve prolapse* are some of the most frequent causes of heart valve surgery *(the valve does not close properly)*. Heart valve surgery may be divided into two categories: *replacement* and *repair.* While a damaged valve can be repaired, a damaged valve must be removed and replaced with an artificial valve in a valve replacement. The amount of the valve's damage and the patient's general condition will determine which operation is performed. A cardiovascular surgeon and anesthesiologist are two members of the highly competent surgical team needed for the difficult operation of heart valve surgery. Usually, general anesthesia is used during the procedure, and the patient must recuperate in the hospital for several days. Patients will need to take drugs after surgery to control any pain or discomfort and to avoid blood clots. Generally, individuals with damaged or unhealthy heart valves may benefit greatly from heart valve surgery. However, there are hazards associated with surgery, and patients should carefully weigh those risks and advantages before having the treatment.

Chapter 5

Alternate Heart Treatments

Herbal remedies for heart disease

Heart disease is a serious condition that requires medical attention and treatment. While some herbal remedies may help with certain aspects of heart health, they should not be used as a replacement for conventional medical care. Always consult with your doctor before starting any new herbal remedies, *especially if you have a heart condition or are taking medication.*

(Garlic) Garlic has been shown to have cardiovascular benefits, including reducing blood pressure and cholesterol levels.

(Hawthorn) Hawthorn is a plant that has been used for centuries to treat heart conditions. It may help to lower blood pressure and improve blood flow to the heart.

(Turmeric) Turmeric contains a compound called curcumin, which has anti-inflammatory properties and may help to improve heart health by reducing inflammation in the body.

(Green tea) Green tea contains catechins, which are antioxidants that may help to reduce the risk of heart disease by protecting the heart and blood vessels.

(Omega-3 fatty acids) Omega-3 fatty acids, found in fatty fish such as salmon, may help to lower

triglycerides and reduce the risk of heart disease. Again, it's important to speak with your doctor before using any herbal remedies for heart disease, as they may interact with medications or have other adverse effects

Heart failure and mindfulness-based interventions

Chronic heart failure reduces the heart's capacity to pump blood efficiently. It may cause signs and symptoms including exhaustion, breathing difficulties, and fluid retention in the body. Although mindfulness and meditation may not be able to treat heart failure, they can offer several advantages that might help individuals who already have the illness live better overall. Stress reduction is one of the main advantages of mindfulness and meditation. Reducing stress can assist improve overall heart health because it is a typical trigger for the symptoms of heart failure.

Deep breathing and body scanning are two mindfulness practices that can help relax the mind and lessen tension and anxiety. Moreover, mindfulness and meditation can aid in enhancing the quality of sleep, which is crucial for those with heart failure. Lack of sleep can raise levels of stress hormones and inflammation, which can worsen the signs and symptoms of heart failure.

Using mindfulness practices can make it easier for people to go to sleep and stay asleep for longer periods, improving their overall health. Lastly, practicing mindfulness and meditation might help you feel better emotionally. Living with heart failure can be difficult, and depressive, anxious, and melancholy sensations are often. Those who practice meditation and mindfulness might have a more optimistic outlook, which can improve their emotional well-being and feeling of well-being. It's crucial to understand that mindfulness and meditation cannot take the place of medical treatment for heart failure. For people suffering from the disease, however, including these techniques in a thorough treatment plan can have several advantages. *When starting a meditation or mindfulness practice,* it's crucial to see a healthcare professional, just as with any new exercise or wellness regimen.

Chapter 6

Resources and Assistance for Heart Health

Heart sufferers' support groups

There are several support groups for cardiac patients, both offline and online.

(U.S. Heart Association) Patients and caregivers can connect with others who are going through comparable situations through the

"*Support Network*," a support network offered by the **American Heart Association**. They provide peer-to-peer help, online forums, and communities for discussion.

Repaired hearts Support for heart patients and their families is offered through the nationwide nonprofit group **Mended Hearts.** In addition to hospital visits and educational resources, they provide nearby support groups.

(WomenHeart) WomenHeart is a national nonprofit that specializes in helping women who have heart disease.

They provide opportunities for advocacy, informational resources, and online support groups.

(America's Heart Support) A nonprofit group called Heart Support of America offers assistance and information to people with heart disease and their families.

They provide a free helpline, neighborhood support groups, and informational resources.

(Meetup) is an online community that links people with similar interests. On Meetup, you can look for neighborhood heart disease support groups to get in touch with people nearby.

Heart rehab facilities Heart sufferers may find cardiac rehab facilities to be quite helpful. They provide education, support groups, and exercise programs.

It's important to keep in mind that support groups can differ in format, subject matter, and level of excellence. It's worthwhile to investigate various options to determine which one best meets your needs.

Information on heart health is available online.

For information on heart health, there are several internet sites accessible.

(American Heart Association (AHA) The AHA website offers details on heart health, cardiovascular conditions, risk factors, and lifestyle modifications that might lower the risk of heart disease.

(**Mayo Clinic**) The Mayo Clinic website provides in-depth information about heart health, including signs and symptoms, causes, diagnosis, and therapy.

(**National Heart, Lung, and Blood Institute**)Information about heart health, including prevention, diagnosis, treatment, and research on heart disease, is available on the NHLBI website.

(*Center for Disease Prevention and Control (CDC)* The CDC website provides details on heart disease, risk factors, and mitigation measures.

(*WebMD*) WebMD is a well-known website for health information that covers a variety of health issues, including heart health.

*(**HeartHub for Patients**)* HeartHub is an online service made available by the AHA that provides data on heart disease, tips for maintaining a healthy lifestyle, and instruments and resources for managing heart health.

*(**MedlinePlus**)* A service of the National Library of Medicine, MedlinePlus offers details on a variety of medical subjects, including heart health. It is crucial to remember that even

while these sites offer insightful information, it is always advisable to seek the assistance of a healthcare expert for specific medical guidance.

*Advice on how to live your life after a heart attack

Although managing life after a heart attack might be difficult, it is possible to lead a healthy and full life with the right care and attention. Here are some guidelines for coping with life after a heart attack.

obey your doctor's instructions, You'll most likely receive a treatment plan from your doctor that entails prescription drugs, lifestyle modifications, and follow-up visits. To guarantee the finest outcome, it's crucial to closely adhere to their instructions. Future cardiac issues may be avoided by adopting a healthy lifestyle. Maintain a heart-healthy diet, engage in regular exercise, abstain from smoking and binge drinking, and control your stress. To help stop more heart damage and regulate your symptoms, it's critical to take the medicine as directed by your doctor. A supervised exercise and education program called cardiac rehabilitation is intended to aid in the recovery process after a heart attack. It can lower your chance of developing future cardiac issues and make you feel better physically and mentally. You can manage the mental and physical difficulties of life after a heart attack by having a solid support system. Get in touch with loved ones, friends, and those who may inspire and uplift you. Learning more about heart health might make it easier for you to comprehend and control your symptoms. Attend support groups or seminars, see your physician, and read information from reliable sources. Maintain a record of your symptoms and any changes to your condition, and let your doctor know about them. This can assist in identifying possible issues early on and avert consequences.

Although recovering after a heart attack requires time and effort, you may live a healthy and full life with the correct treatment and support

Conclusion

Aim for a strong heart and a joyous existence.

A happy and satisfying existence depends on a healthy heart. You may take several steps to strengthen your heart and raise your likelihood of living a long and healthy life. Frequent exercise increases blood flow, lowers blood pressure, and strengthens the heart muscle, all of which lessen the risk of heart disease. A heart-healthy diet should be balanced and full of fruits, vegetables, whole grains, lean meats, and healthy fats. Obesity or being overweight might raise your chance of developing heart disease. This risk can be decreased by maintaining a healthy weight through food and exercise. A significant risk factor for heart disease is smoking. Your heart health can be considerably improved by not smoking or by never beginning. High blood pressure and other heart-related issues can result from persistent stress. Using appropriate coping mechanisms for stress, such as meditation, physical activity, or quality time with loved ones, might lessen the negative effects on your heart. You may enhance your heart health and raise your chances of having a long and happy life by implementing these routines into your everyday life. Start looking for your heart now by keeping in mind that even tiny

adjustments over time can result
in significant gains.